THE SURROGATE'S TABLE: HEALTHY RECIPES FOR PREGNANCY SUPPORT

Explore a culinary journey of wellness with recipes crafted to nourish and sustain surrogate mothers through their incredible journey

Roland D. Ward

Chapter One

Nutritional Needs for Surrogate Mothers

The impact of nutrition is enormous when surrogate women begin out on their goal to carry a child to term. In this chapter, we review the nutrients essential for a healthy surrogacy experience and provide feasible suggestions for reaching perfect nutrition as we dig thoroughly into the crucial role that nutrition plays in boosting the health and well-being of surrogate mothers. An act of altruistic love, surrogacy asks for immense physical and mental endurance. Supporting the surrogate mother's health throughout the pregnancy relies crucially on providing proper nutrients. The body changes drastically from the beginning of conception until the final seconds of birth, and to support the growth and development of the baby, more critical nutrients must be ingested.

Meeting these elevated dietary needs, however, may be challenging, especially in light of the mental and physical demands of pregnancy. It could be challenging for surrogate mothers to keep to a balanced diet because of their sickness, culinary aversions, and desires. The likelihood of gestational diabetes and other disorders connected to pregnancy further underlines the significance of eating properly.

It could be challenging for surrogate mothers to keep to a balanced diet because of their sickness, culinary aversions, and desires. The likelihood of gestational diabetes and other disorders connected to pregnancy further underlines the significance of eating properly.

Dietitians and obstetricians, among other medical professionals, may provide surrogate mothers individualized dietary guidance and help as they manage these challenges. Planning meals, incorporating a variety of foods strong in nutrients, and drinking lots of water are key techniques for assuring appropriate nutrition all along the surrogacy process.

Pregnancy-related mental health is substantially benefited by healthy eating in addition to physical health. Emotions experienced by surrogate moms could be anything from pleased and enthusiastic to frightened and freaked out. A diet abundant in fruits, vegetables, healthful grains, and lean meats may help to balance mood, lessen stress, and enhance overall mental wellness.

In the end, surrogate mothers may optimize their health and well-being and ensure a safe and successful surrogacy experience for the intended parents as well as themselves by giving nutrition first priority and selecting appropriately. Remembering the significant effect that diet has on the wonder of life and the requirement of feeding both body and spirit as we begin our exploration into healthy recipes for pregnancy support.

Chapter Two
Building a Kitchen That Is Surrogate-Friendly

Building a kitchen that is hospitable to surrogates is a critical first step in assuring their health and welfare throughout their pregnancy. We analyze in this chapter the major components of a kitchen that is both useful and nutritious, from meal preparation organization to storing required commodities.

A kitchen that is surrogate-friendly has a selection of nutrient-dense goods on hand to make nutritious meals and snacks easier to prepare. A balanced diet is based on fresh fruits and vegetables, whole grains, lean proteins, and healthy fats, which give critical nutrients to the growing baby as well as the surrogate mother.

Give fresh, natural food first priority when stocking your kitchen above processed and packaged foods. Whenever you can, purchase seasonal food; it is generally more flavorful, fresher, and less costly. Select whole grains—including brown rice, quinoa, and oats—over processed grains, which have lost all of their nutritious value, including white rice and white bread.

Excellent sources of iron and required amino acids include lean proteins like chicken, fish, tofu, beans, and lentils; nutritious fats like those in avocados, nuts, seeds, and olive oil are important for hormone production and brain development. Rich in calcium and protein, dairy foods including milk, cheese, and yoghurt help both foetal development and bone health.

A surrogate-friendly kitchen should be filled with good ingredients as well as the tools and technology essential to rapidly create healthy meals. To ease and enjoy meal preparation, make an investment in superior cookware, knives, and utensils. Think about acquiring a food processor or blender to produce sauces, soups, and smoothies and an Instant Pot or slow cooker for simple meal preparation.

Keeping a kitchen surrogate-friendly involves organisation. Keep nutritional staples in your freezer, refrigerator, and pantry, and use labels and clear containers to keep track of items. Put regularly used objects in easy reach and less often used things in readily accessible but out-of-the-way areas to improve efficiency in your kitchen.

Building a surrogate-friendly kitchen also involves thoughtful food planning. Spend some time each week planning your meals and snacks, considering your schedule, food choices, and nutritional needs. When at all practicable, prepare meals in advance, batch cooking and freezing portions for later use.

You may make your surrogacy experience effective by constructing a kitchen that is favourable to surrogates. This will allow you to promote your overall health and well-being and to keep to a balanced diet. One wonderful supper at a time, you can nourish your body and spirit with the necessary ingredients, equipment, and preparation.

Chapter Three
Breakfasts to Energise Your Day

There is good reason why breakfast is sometimes regarded as the most significant meal of the day. It provides your body with the nutrients it needs to fasten metabolism, maintain steady blood sugar levels, and provide you with energy throughout morning. For surrogate parents in particular, breakfast sets the tone for the rest of the day and supplies essential sustenance for both mother and child. This chapter offers lots of tasty, wholesome breakfast ideas to help surrogate parents feel rested and invigorated before their amazing trip. Overnight Oats: A flexible, wholesome breakfast option that may be made to your specifications. Add the Greek yoghurt, chia seeds, honey or maple syrup, and your choice of milk (vegan or cow). Beat in the seeds and nuts and fresh fruit. Adorn with vanilla essence, chocolate powder, or cinnamon. Cold nights should be spent, and start your day with a substantial meal. Dispensing bowls Smoothie bowls are a refreshing and substantial morning alternative that combine the ease of a smoothie with the fullness of a bowl. Blend your selected fruits, leafy greens, protein powder and liquid base (such as almond milk or coconut water) until smooth and creamy. For added flavour and texture, top a bowl of smoothie with fresh fruit, nuts, seeds, and granola. Smoothie bowls are tasty, full of antioxidants, vitamins, and minerals that enhance overall health and well-being.

Vegetable Omelette: Packed full of protein and fibre, omelettes are a delicious and filling breakfast food that will keep you going till lunch. Beat the eggs, herbs, salt, and pepper with a tiny bit of milk. Spoon mixture into pan; cook until set. Top with cheese and the veggies of your choice (tomatoes, onions, bell peppers, and spinach, for instance). Fry, turning the omelette about halfway through, until the cheese has melted and the veggies are soft. For a full and healthy dinner, serve with whole grain bread or pieces of avocado.

Whole grain pancakes are a pleasant and healthy meal choice that can be made ahead of time and kept in the refrigerator for easy warming on busy mornings. Add the baking powder, salt, and sweetener—like maple syrup or honey—to the whole wheat flour. In an other dish, beat the eggs, milk, and vanilla essence. Simply stir the dry ingredients into the wet components. Fry the pancakes on a hot griddle till golden brown and cooked through for a filling and healthy breakfast. Present with honey, Greek yoghurt and fresh fruit.

Quick and simple, avocado toast offers the right amount of protein, carbohydrates, and good fats to keep you feeling full and energised. Drizzle chopped avocado, lemon juice and sea salt over a golden-brown slice of whole grain bread. Add scrambled eggs, microgreens or chopped tomatoes for more taste and protein. Avocado toast feels great and is high in enzymes, minerals, and vitamins that improve general health and well-being.

Chia seed pudding is a great, creamy breakfast choice and keeps well in the refrigerator for easy grab-and-go dinners. To dairy or veggie milk, add chia seeds, along with flavourings like vanilla essence or chocolate powder, and for sweetness, honey or maple syrup. Stirring till thick and creamy, chill for four hours or over night. Over the chia seed pudding, spread some fresh fruit, nuts and seeds to provide a bit more taste and structure. High in vitamins, omega-3 fatty acids, and protein, chia seed cream benefits general and gut health. It feels wonderful too.

Greek parfait made with yoghurt : Easy to modify to suit your dietary requirements and tastes, this filling and healthful breakfast meal tastes great. Making a beautiful and tasty morning parfait in a glass or container, layer fresh fruit, oats, almonds, and seeds. While fresh fruit supplies vitamins, minerals, and antioxidants to improve general health, Greek yoghurt is high in protein and probiotics, which help the immune system and digestive health. Granola, almonds and seeds provide you the crunch and texture you need along with fibre and good fats to keep you full until lunch.

The Breakfast Burrito: For hectic mornings, they are simple to reheat and freezer-safe. Top scrambled eggs, black beans, chopped veggies, and shredded cheese on whole grain tortillas; shape into burritos and cover securely with foil. Up to a month after they were frozen, reheat the burritos through in the microwave or oven. For a substantial and revitalising meal that will keep you going all morning, serve the breakfast burritos with Greek yoghurt, avocado, and salsa.

Chapter Four
Nourishing Lunches for Long-Term Energy

Lunch is important as it gives surrogate moms a vitamin and energy boost to get them through the afternoon. This chapter covers a variety of filling lunch choices meant to feed the body and promote general comfort and health while surrogacy is being done. A quinoa salad and roast veggies meal is filling and active, with just the right mix of vitamins, carbs, and protein. Top the rice with red onion, zucchini, cherry tomatoes and roasted red peppers after cooking it according to the package directions. Swirl the salad with the honey basic sauce, balsamic vinegar, Dijon mustard, and olive oil mixture. Grind in the thyme, basil, and parsley. A tasty and nutrient-dense quinoa salad with roasted veggies will support general health and well-being. Stir-Fry Brown Rice Vegetables This quick and simple supper may be changed to meet your health needs. In a hot pan, stir-fry until crisp-tender your best vegetables: broccoli, carrots, snap peas, bell peppers, and mushrooms. Spice things up with a little soy sauce, garlic, and ginger. For a full, high-fiber, vitamin and mineral-rich lunch, spoon the stir-fry over cooked brown rice. Delicious and full of great fats and plant-based nutrition to support general health and fitness is veggie stir-fry with brown rice.

An excellent lunchtime protein-rich choice that provides important nutrients to support muscle growth and repair is the turkey and avocado wrap. Ladder pieces of roasted turkey breast, lettuce, tomato, onion, and sprouts over mashed avocado in a whole grain tortilla. For a quick and easy morning to go, tightly roll and slice in half the tortilla. Made with turkey and avocado, this delicious, high-nutrient wrap supports general health and well-being.

Dressing for salmon salad with lemon and dill A delicious and healthy meal on hot days is salmon salad with a lemon-dill sauce. Whether grilled or baked, well cooked fish should flake and be served with mixed greens, avocado, cherry tomatoes, cucumber and red onion. Stir in a sauce made from chopped dill, Dijon mustard, honey, and fresh lemon juice. Delicious and high in vitamins and omega-3 fatty acids to support heart health and general health is salmon salad with a lemon-dill sauce.

Mondays are ideal days to have the filling and hearty lunch of quesadillas made with black beans and sweet potatoes. Add cooked black beans, chopped red onion, cilantro, cumin, and chilli powder to sweet potato cubes and bake until soft. Spoon mix of black beans and sweet potatoes onto whole grain tortillas; cover with another tortilla and shredded cheese. Once cut and crisped on a hot grill, the quesadillas are best served with salsa, guacamole, and Greek yoghurt for dipping. Sweet potato and black bean quesadillas are delicious and packed with vitamins, minerals, and protein to support general health and fitness.

Mediterranean Chickpea Salad: This sort of light and cool dinner is great for the summer heat wave. Add the feta, cherry tomatoes, cucumber, red onion, cooked chickpeas, and Kalamata olives to a big bowl. Toss the salad with a simple sauce of olive oil, red wine vinegar, garlic, herbs, and lemon juice.

For a delicious, high-nutrient meal that will promote general health and well-being, serve the Mediterranean chickpea salad over mixed veggies.

On cold days, a filling and tasty lunch is vegetable and bean soup. Put the chopped carrots, celery, onion, garlic, and canned tomatoes into a big pot. Cook, covered, until tastes have mixed and veggies are soft. Whisk in the black pepper, bay leaves, thyme, and rosemary. Present warm and with a bit of whole grain bread for dipping. A tasty and high-protein, high-fiber meal that improves general health and well-being is veggie and lentil soup.

A very full and normal lunch choice is grilled chicken Caesar salad. Cook the chicken breast fully, then slice it thinly and put it on crisp lettuce leaves. Anchovies, garlic, Dijon mustard, Worcestershire sauce, lemon juice and olive oil should all be added to the salad. For even more taste and crunch, top with more Parmesan cheese and croutons. Delicious and high in protein, vitamins, and minerals to support general health and well-being is grilled chicken Caesar salad.

These all-inclusive lunch plans are just a few of the many delicious and healthy meals surrogate moms may have throughout their pregnancy. Giving their bodies and general health and well-being first importance, surrogate moms may ensure a happy and safe surrogacy experience for the intended parents as well as for themselves.

Chapter Five
Nutrient-Dense Meals for Surrogate Mothers

Dinner is a moment to refill, refresh, and recover after a hard day of travel. It is not just a meal. Dinner is even more important to surrogate moms because it is a chance to feed the valuable life growing inside of them as well as themselves. Here in this chapter, we explore a world of healthy meals meant to keep surrogate moms active and alive during their incredible trip. A blend of tastes and nutrients, grilled chicken with roasted veggies and rice offers a well-balanced mix of protein, carbs, and important vitamins and minerals. For delicious cooking, prepare chicken breasts in a blend of olive oil, lemon juice, garlic, and herbs. In the meantime, sprinkle a variety of bright veggies—like cherry tomatoes, zucchini, and bell peppers—in olive oil, salt, and pepper, then cook until soft and toasted. For a taste and freshness burst, top the grilled chicken and roasted veggies with fluffy rice and fresh herbs. A filling and cosy meal choice that honours the earthy depth of lentils and veggies is vegetarian lentil shepherd's pie. Simmer cooked lentils in a delicious tomato-based sauce spiced with rosemary and thyme, along with onions, carrots, celery and mushrooms. Top the lentil mixture in a baking dish with creamy mashed potatoes, and bake until bubbly and brown. The end result is a filling and healthy dinner high in fibre, plant-based protein, and a range of vitamins and minerals to support general health and fitness. Salmon and Asparagus Foil packages: These easy-to-make, mess-free supper packages need little planning or cleanup. Lay out the fish pieces and the cleaned asparagus stalks on separate metal foil sheets. Drizzle with olive oil and season with lemon slices, salt, and pepper. Tightly seal the foil bags, then bake or grill the asparagus until it is crisp and the salmon is crispy. A wonderful and light dinner high in protein, vitamins, and heart-healthy omega-3 fatty acids is the result, ideal for feeding body and mind. Peas and Parmesan Mushroom Risotto: Rich umami taste and a creamy texture make this elegant yet easy supper dish enthral the senses. After sautéing chopped mushrooms in butter and garlic until fragrant and golden brown, add Arborio rice and toast just till gently toasted. Stirring continually, gently pour in hot chicken or veggie broth until the rice is smooth and soft. For a burst of colour and freshness, stir in grated Parmesan cheese and frozen peas until cooked through. This rich dinner feeds and soothes the body and soul at the same time.

Thai-Styled Tofu Peanut Noodles: This bright and delicious supper dish transports the palate to the streets of Bangkok. As directed on the box, cook rice noodles. Toss them with a creamy peanut sauce consisting of peanut butter, soy sauce, lime juice, ginger, garlic, and a little amount of honey. For colour, crunch and nutritional depth, add pan-fried tofu pieces and a variety of fresh vegetables like carrots, bell peppers and snap peas. For a particularly light and flavorful topping, chop up some lime leaves, parsley and peanuts.

This filling and cosy dinner option, Vegetable and Chickpea Curry with Basmati Rice, nurtures the body and spirit. In coconut oil, sautée onions, garlic, ginger and spices (turmeric, cumin, and curry powder) until aromatic and golden brown. Stir in chopped potatoes, carrots, and broccoli to the cooked beans and creamy coconut milk. Simmer until vegetables are tender and flavours combine for a satisfying, high-protein, high-fiber dinner; serve hot over fragrant basmati rice.

Chapter Six
Indulgent Snacks for Mothers Who Surrogate

Snacking not only relieves hunger but also gives the chance to refuel the body, boost energy, and spend some time on oneself. Because surrogate moms have to juggle the demands of pregnancy with everyday tasks, smart eating is critical to their health and well-being. This chapter studies a range of rich treats meant to please the taste and boost the soul on this amazing trip.

A classic that never goes out of style is a Greek yoghurt spread with granola and fresh berries. Arrange a bright collection of fresh berries, including raspberries, blueberries, and strawberries, over crisp granola for a symphony of tastes and textures. A blast of sweetness and vitamins from the berries and creamy, tart base rich in protein and probiotics from the yoghurt. For crunch and nutrition, top with a sprinkle of oats, and you have a substantial, nutrient-dense breakfast.

Rich and healthy, dark chocolate-dipped banana slices fill appetites without losing nutrients. Just slice ripe bananas into pieces and dip each one halfway into hot dark chocolate. To add even more taste and texture, arrange the coated banana slices on a parchment paper-lined baking sheet and sprinkle with shredded coconut or chopped nuts. After the chocolate sets, freeze it and then have this guilt-free, antioxidant- and fibre-rich treat.

Handcrafted at Home Journey To fit individual nutritional needs and tastes, mix with nuts, seeds, and dried fruit. Blend a range of nuts—including cashews, walnuts, and almonds—with seeds like sunflower and pumpkin for a base rich in nutrients. For sweetness and chewiness, add dried fruit such as apricots, cranberries or raisins. Blend in a sprinkle of dark chocolate chips for even more richness. Pack each serving—which offers a substantial mix of protein, healthy fats, and antioxidants—in sealed bags for easy eating on-the-go.

Avocado toast is given a wonderful new twist by the creamy hummus and lush cherry tomato. Mash avocado over whole grain bread, then generously top with hummus for extra flavour and nutrients. Halved cherry tomatoes provide a burst of sweetness and freshness to this nutrient-dense and delicious snack. Then sprinkle with crushed black pepper and sea salt.

Cucumber slices are raised to refined appetiser level when topped with delicate smoked salmon and herb cream cheese. Spread a thin layer of herbed cream cheese over cucumber rounds and top with a slice of smoked salmon for a taste blast of creamy, sour, and salty. A cold and rich snack great for a quiet day or gathering, top with fresh dill or chives for a pop of colour.

These caprese skewers mix fresh mozzarella, cherry tomatoes and basil for a standard bite-sized taste of Italy. Thread cheese balls, cherry tomatoes and little basil leaves onto wooden skewers for a delicious and visually appealing snack. Drizzle with balsamic glaze or spread flake sea salt over for a taste depth that will wow.

Apple slices dipped in creamy almond butter and a dusting of cinnamon become a snack that will make you want more. For a contenting blend of sweetness, creaminess, and crunch, spread almond butter over apple slices. For a warm, reassuring flavour that brings back memories of freshly made apple pie, dust with ground cinnamon. This makes a filling and healthful snack that works well any time of day. Spiced Roasted Chickpeas: Easy to prepare and really filling, roasted chickpeas are crunchy and tasty. Toss cooked chickpeas with olive oil and your preferred seasonings, such garlic powder, cumin, and paprika. Spread onto a baking pan and roast until golden brown, crispy perfection. Chill before using as a high-protein snack that is great for topping salads for crunch or for snacking on the go. These decadent nibbles represent only a small portion of the many delectable and nourishing alternatives open to surrogate moms. Surrogate moms may fuel their bodies, sate their appetites, and celebrate the joy of eating healthily during this amazing journey by accepting the pleasure of mindful snacking and selecting healthy products.

Grilled Vegetable and Hummus Wraps: Honouring the wealth of the season, these wraps are a light and cool supper choice. After cooking a variety of bright veggies, including eggplant, bell peppers, and zucchini, till soft and browned, top whole grain wraps with a generous amount of hummus. For extra depth and taste, top the grilled veggies with fresh leaves, sliced avocado, and feta cheese. Perfect for warm summer nights, roll up the wraps firmly and cut in two for a filling and healthy dinner.

Edamame and Sesame Dressed Soba Noodle Salad: This light and refreshing supper dish is both delicious and nourishing. After cooking soba noodles per the package directions, throw with chopped scallions, shredded carrots, thinly sliced cucumbers, and steamed edamame. Toss to coat after drizzling with a tart sesame dressing prepared with soy sauce, rice vinegar, sesame oil, and sugar. For a taste-bud-teasing explosion of flavour and texture, garnish with fresh cilantro and toasted sesame seeds. The world of gastronomic alternatives open to surrogate mothers is much larger than these healthful meal selections. Surrogate moms may feed their bodies, please their senses, and enjoy the pleasure of eating healthily on their amazing journey by putting nutrient-dense foods, vivid flavours, and inventive cooking techniques first. This chapter provides a rich tapestry of meal options, each expertly designed to provide surrogate moms the energy and contentment they need to flourish. These recipes, which range from colourful salads to savoury stews, reflect the goodness of whole foods and the pleasure of dining with loved ones. We are going to go on a gastronomic journey that will please the senses, nourishe the body, and uplift the spirit.

Chapter Seven

**Desserts to Savour: Delightful Treats for
Mothers Who Surrogate**

Desserts have a particular place in our hearts since they are happy, celebratory, and comforting times as well as pleasures. Desserts give surrogate moms, who set out on a road of love and kindness, a well-earned chance to enjoy the pleasure of life. Here in this chapter, we dive into a delicious selection of desserts meant to fulfil the hunger and boost the spirit on this amazing journey.

Fruit Salad with Honey-Lime Dressing: This bright and cool dessert choice honours the natural wealth of fresh fruits. Combine in a big dish a bright mix of seasonal fruits, including mango, pineapple, kiwi, and strawberries. Drizzle with a simple sauce of lime juice, honey, and a little salt; toss just enough to coat. For a splash of colour and brightness, top with fresh mint leaves to make a light and healthy treat great for warm weather days.

Berries Dipped in Dark Chocolate: A traditional pleasure that never goes out of style are dark chocolate-dipped strawberries. After wrapping ripe strawberries with melted dark chocolate, place them on a baking sheet lined with parchment paper. Enjoy this guilt-free, vitamin- and mineral-rich treat after letting the chocolate firm. To give these delicious pieces of joy even more grace, sprinkle with shredded coconut or chopped nuts before the chocolate sets.

Berries and Almonds Frozen Yoghurt Bark: This delicious and refreshing treat is as beautiful as it is healthy. After smoothing and evening out Greek yoghurt on a baking sheet lined with parchment paper, top with chopped almonds and fresh berries (like black, blue, and raspberries) for a touch of crunch and taste. Break into pieces after freezing until hard, then enjoy as a cool, creamy treat that will please sweet tooths without losing health.

Naturally sweetened and dairy-free, banana lovely cream with peanut butter swirl is a rich and delicious dessert choice. Ripe bananas are frozen till hard, then mixed until smooth and creamy, if necessary adding a little almond milk to get the right consistency. For a rich and delicious taste, swirl in a good dollop of peanut butter. Serve right away for a delicious and guilt-free treat that will please any sweet stomach.

Mixed Berry Chia Seed Pudding: This healthy and filling dessert is ideal for treating yourself to a guilt-free pleasure. In a jar or dish, mix chia seeds with your favourite milk—almond, coconut, or cashew milk, for example—and then add a little honey or maple syrup to taste. Chia seeds will soak fluids and thicken into a pudding-like consistency if kept over night. For an antioxidant- and color-packed explosion, serve topped with a mix of fresh berries, such raspberries, blueberries, and strawberries.

A warm and cosy dessert choice for chilly fall nights are baked apples with cinnamon-oat crumble. After coreing and arranging apples in a baking dish, stuff each hole with a mix of brown sugar, cinnamon, rolled oats, and a little butter or coconut oil. For a pleasant, filling and healthy treat, bake until the apples are soft and the crumble is golden and crunchy. Serve warm with a scoop of vanilla ice cream or a dollop of Greek yoghurt.

Tropical and rich, coconut mango rice pudding is the ideal food to sate sweet tooths with a bit of the unusual.

For a taste and sweetness explosion, throw in chopped mango after cooking rice in coconut milk until creamy and soft. For extra warmth and flavour depth, top warm or cold servings with toasted coconut flakes and ground cardamom or cinnamon. Every mouthful of this luscious and reassuring treat will take the taste senses to a tropical paradise. Lemon Blueberry Cheesccake Bars: These rich, tart dessert bars are ideal for treating yourself to a little sweet treat. For flavour and sweetness explosions, mix in fresh blueberries after smoothing and creamying cream cheese, Greek yoghurt, lemon zest, and honey. Spoon mixture over graham cracker crust, bake until done, then chill until solid before cutting into bars and serving. Any event will be enhanced by these delicious, creamy cheesecake bars. These delicacies are evidence of the richness and happiness life has to provide. Through the acceptance of the enjoyment of decadent foods and the selection of healthful ingredients, surrogate mothers can nourishe their bodies, uplift their spirits, and enjoy every second of this amazing journey. We have looked at many sweets in this chapter that are meant to entice the palate and uplift the spirit. Fruity delights and creamy indulgences, these sweets are guaranteed to provide surrogate moms moments of happiness and fulfilment while they negotiate the pleasures and difficulties of

pregnancy. Enjoy a piece of sweetness and
the wonder of dessert time, then.

Chapter Eight
Responsible Approaches to Surrogates'
Health

A very transforming experience, surrogacy affects not just the physical but also the mind, body, and soul. Through an examination of the advantages of mindfulness and self-care techniques for surrogate mothers, we provide a comprehensive approach to wellness that supports the full person in this chapter.

Benefits of Mindfulness Meditation A technique for promoting inner tranquilly and present awareness, mindfulness meditation gives surrogate moms a potent instrument for stress reduction and improved overall health. By routine quiet reflection, breathing exercises, and uncritical observation of thoughts and emotions, surrogate mothers may develop a sense of peace and serenity that accompanies them through the highs and lows of the surrogacy process.

Yoga Bends and Strengthens With its all-encompassing approach of movement, breathing, and mindfulness, yoga offers surrogate mothers a potent means of strengthening their bodies, promoting inner calm, and enhancing their physical health. Whether they do gentle hatha yoga, flowing vinyasa sequences, or soothing yin yoga, yoga feeds surrogate moms on the physical, emotional, and spiritual levels. Throughout the surrogacy process, yoga maintains women in balance and harmony.

Writing for Reflection and Personal Development Writing provides surrogate moms with a sacred and secure place to process their ideas, emotions, and experiences. Written down, surrogate moms might develop personally and become more resilient and self-aware in the process.

Joy-Promoting Gratitude Exercises: Surrogate moms have the ability to turn their attention from the somewhat challenging or unpleasant aspects of their life to the wonderful and wonderful ones. Every day people may develop a profound feeling of pleasure, contentment, and gratitude that nourishes the soul and elevates the spirit by taking the time to consider the tiny and large blessings that surround them—from the support of loved ones to the wonder of new life.

Stress-Reduction Breathing Exercises Deliberate breathing exercises help surrogate moms relax, reduce tension, and enhance their overall health fast and easily.

Surrogate moms may take advantage of the body's natural ability for self-regulation and healing via deep belly breathing, alternative nostril breathing, or breath awareness meditation, thereby reestablishing balance to the mind, body, and soul.

Nature Walks to Ground and Reconnect Surrogate moms who spend time in nature are better able to ground themselves in the present, reestablish a connection with the earth, and find tranquilly again. Whether they are climbing in the mountains, enjoying a leisurely walk in the park, or simply resting under a tree and listening to the sounds of nature, the natural environment may provide surrogate mothers comfort and support in its beauty and wisdom.

Joyful Expression for Self-Awarenes Surrogate moms may find great psychological benefit in writing, dancing, singing, or sketching. Surrogate parents may access a rich source of inspiration and understanding and may uncover new aspects of themselves and their journey in the process by letting themselves to explore their creativity without expectation or critique.

Contacting the Community to Get Support and Empowerment

Surrogate mothers may benefit much from establishing relationships with other surrogate mothers and other surrogacy community members in terms of empowerment, validation, and support. With like-minded people, surrogate moms might feel less alone and be more equipped to manage the intricacies of the surrogacy process with grace, boldness, and resilience.

By offering a whole approach to health that nourishes their body, mind, and spirit, these mindful techniques help surrogate mothers to bravely, elegantly, and compassionately welcome every aspect of their surrogacy journey.

Conclusion
Finally, accepting the surrogacy journey with grace and thankfulness

It is obvious as we draw to a close this tour through the world of The Surrogate's Table: Healthy Recipes for Pregnancy Support that surrogacy is a deep and life-changing journey of love, sacrifice, and empowerment rather than just a physical procedure. We have looked at many ways that surrogate mothers can support their bodies, brains, and souls as they set out on this amazing journey throughout this book.

Every page in this book has served as a tribute to the bravery, fortitude, and beauty of surrogate mothers everywhere, from the healthy recipes created to promote the best possible health and well-being throughout pregnancy to the thoughtful techniques created to foster inner calm. We have honoured the special relationship between surrogate mothers and the families they help build, praised the pleasure of sharing healthful meals with loved ones, and accepted the potential of mindfulness and self-care in enhancing general wellness.

Deep appreciation is at the core of it all, for the gift of new life, for the support of loved ones, and for the chance to participate in something very remarkable. Love, connection, and deep personal development are among the incalculable benefits of the adventure that is surrogacy, but it also requires bravery, tenacity, and unflinching dedication.

You surrogate moms represent the highest kind of love, compassion, and selflessness. You are the unsung heroes that realise aspirations, give hope to those in need, and represent the real meaning of selflessness for the benefit of others. While not an easy path, it is one that is rich in grace, fortitude, and deep significance that will never be forgotten by everyone who is lucky enough to be touched by your unselfish act of love.

Let us take the lessons discovered, the experiences had, and the love that unites us with us as we say goodbye to these pages and start the next chapter of our lives. Continuing to feed our bodies, minds, and spirits with grace, compassion, and kindness, let us know that we are loved, supported, and much valued at every stage.

Thus, we sincerely thank, admire, and support all of the surrogate mothers who have started this amazing adventure. As you carry on lighting the globe and inspiring us all with your tremendous bravery and compassion, may love fill your hearts, hope elevate your spirits, and grace lead your path.

Many conscious strategies designed to support surrogate mothers in taking care of themselves and living out their surrogacy journey have been explored in this chapter. These methods give surrogate moms a whole approach to health that honors the spirit, body, and mind. They include anything from yoga to mindfulness meditation, gratitude exercises to journaling, breathwork to nature walks, artistic expression to community building. Thus, taking a moment to breathe and connect with the knowledge and resiliency that already resides within of you, remember that you are loved, supported, and highly valued on this incredible surrogacy journey.